Intermittent Fasting (IF)

BY

ISLAM AHMED

Copyright © 2018

Table of Contents

Introduction

What is Intermittent Fasting (IF)?

"Intermittent" is characterized as "happening in sporadic interims". The word fasting is a demonstration in which one avoids a specific action for a particular time of time. Essentially put Intermittent Fasting (IF) is shunning nourishment for a specific day and age.

On the off chance that has two segments

• A fasting period: time interim in which you shun eating
• A sustaining window: time interim in which you are permitted to eat.

What Intermittent Fasting (IF) isn't?

• IF is certainly not an enchantment projectile for weight reduction, you won't lose 10lbs of every multi week. You may anyway make reliable misfortune, for example, 1pound every week.

• IF does not claim to be the best eating routine or the best way to deal with eating less junk food for everybody. In the event that is a disentangled eating routine strategy that works best for the bustling person.

• IF isn't a need. On the off chance that, it similar to each other eating routine is only an apparatus to enable you to lose weight. Consider it another instrument to add to your tool compartment for fat-misfortune. There are a lot of different approaches to get more fit.

For what reason would it be a good idea for you to quick?

Irregular fasting has numerous advantages, here is a couple.

• Lower circulatory strain

• Lower oxidative pressure

• Increased fat consuming

• Increased metabolic rate amid the quick

• Improved craving control

• Improved glucose control

• Improved cardiovascular capacity

Who is this manual for?

This manual is for the individuals who

• Want to take in the fundamental of irregular fasting

• Want to enhance their wellbeing

• Experience a predictable and sensible approach to get more fit.

• Want to cling to an eating regimen and without the issue of being constrained to certain nourishments.

• This manual accept that you have an activity program to go with an IF eat less carbs program. Most extreme fat misfortune can't be accomplished through eating routine alone.

It is a mix of activity and eating regimen that produces greatest fat misfortune. In the event that you don't have an activity program don't fear. An activity program can be as just as running for 30minutes multi day. Any way it ought to be noticed that a very much outlined preparing program that is custom-made towards your objective will create the best outcomes.

The basics for an effective Intermittent Fasting (IF) program

• Dedication

• Determination

• your body

• A decent exercise program

what you needn't

• you won't have to purchase particular sustenance's, eat what you need to however recall control is the key factor.

• You won't require a fitness coach in the event that you are knowledgeable in preparing. On the off chance that you are not you may search out a mentor or counsel the web for data.

• You needn't bother with any shady fat consuming supplements.

Section 1: Basic Dietary Guidelines

The accompanying data can be connected to any eating routine. Before you begin any eating routine it is critical that you acclimate yourself with the nuts and bolts of an eating regimen.

How does weight reduction happen?

Weight reduction is a procedure of being in a caloric deficiency. A caloric shortfall is the point at which you utilize a larger number of calories than you are expending. Weight reduction can't happen without a caloric shortfall. Return and read the last sentence until the point that you have completely gotten a handle on the idea of weight reduction.

Imagine a scenario where I need to put on weight.

Since weight reduction happens when we are not expending enough calories to meet our day by day utilize, at that point weight pick up is the inverse. Weight pick up happens when we surpass our day by day caloric needs therefore the additional calories are put away as fat. On the off chance that you instigate a boost, for example, weight preparing than the additional calories will be utilized to repair and enhance the harmed muscles accordingly expanding your muscles and at last outcomes in you putting on muscle weight.

Saving Muscle

You generally hear individuals saying "I need to get more fit" or "I have to lose some weight" however they never indicate what kind of weight. Muscle adds to your aggregate bodyweight as well, so does water, and your organs et cetera. You could lose 10lbs of muscle, however would you be fulfilled? The right expression is "I need to lose fat". Commonly (fat tissue) is the thing that a great many people are alluding to when they need to shed pounds. Anyway what inescapable occurs mid an eating regimen is muscle misfortune. Here's the reason.

Muscles are calorically costly. Consider it a bank. Say each pound of slender muscle requires 25 calories to maintain. So if 100lbs of your aggregate bodyweight is unadulterated muscle than you have to eat 2,500 calories per day just to keep up your bulk. Say now you need to start eating better so you diminish your calories down 2,300. Presently an issue emerges. You don't have enough calories to keep up your bulk. As yet utilizing the bank similarity, you are currently given two decisions you can auction your muscle (separate muscle tissue to pay for alternate muscles and decrease add up to spending) or you can apply for a new line of credit (separate greasy tissue for additional calories).

In a perfect world you need the last since that is what fat is for right? Fat is to be utilized as vitality when we are in a shortage.

So at that point how does muscle misfortune happen? Muscle misfortune happens when we surpass our advance breaking point. Say our shortfall is presently 1500 calories despite everything we require 2500 calories every day. We wind up down 1000 calories anyway we can just take out a maximum credit of 500 calories from our fat stores. This point of confinement happens in light of the fact that there is a utmost to which fat can be separated. Hence we are power to breakdown a portion of our muscle to pay for the rest. So in conclusion to limit muscle misfortunes dependably decrease your every day calorie needs by little augmentations (200 or 100 calories) with the goal that you don't surpass your advance farthest point. Use a quality preparing project to guarantee that your body understands that your muscles are required.

Are largely calories met?

Truly are calories are equivalent. There is no such thing as great sustenance and awful nourishment just sustenance that are more calorie thick (higher in calories) and nourishment that are bring down in calories. In the event that regardless you have questions about a calorie being a calorie, go read about the teacher who lost 27 pounds while eating just Twinkies.

All calories are equivalent, however are generally nourishments measure up to?

I said before that there aren't such things as great nourishments or awful sustenance's well that was a lie. There are sustenance's that are filled to the overflow with man-made synthetics, for example, high fructose corn syrup. These synthetic concoctions are possibly hurtful and therefore ought to be evaded or kept to a base. When in doubt the closer the nourishment is to its common frame, the better. I am not saying that you can't make the most of your most loved sustenance's however just expressing that the greater part of your eating regimen should comprise of regular nourishments. The advantages of a solid eating routine are interminable yet here are a couple

• Higher vitality levels

• Better disposition

Less danger of maladies

• Stronger invulnerable framework

• Healthier skin

• Stronger bones

• Longer life

Macronutrients and Caloric Maintenance

I won't dive excessively into this theme as there is an abundance of data on the web and it would be outside the extent of this manual. So look at this as a short prologue to macronutrients.

Macronutrients are protein, starches, and lipids (fats).

Protein:

If you are a genuine weight lifter or a competitor then you ought to know about the significance of protein. Proteins are the building square of muscle and any guide in recuperation after an instructional course. Of the three (carbs, fats, and protein) protein is the most vital. Protein can be found in meats, dairy, nuts, and vegetables (beans). The general manager for any competitor is 1 gram of protein for every pound of bodyweight. For instance on the off chance that you weigh 150lbs than you should endeavor to eat 150 grams of protein for every day. Every gram of protein is identical to roughly 4 calories

Starches:

 Carbohydrates are your body's fundamental wellspring of vitality. The lion's share of your day by day calories will come as starches. Starches come in two noteworthy structures, sugars and starches. Sugars are effectively processed and in this way enter the circulatory system promptly. Starches require a significant stretch of time to process and are regularly put away in the muscles as glycogen. Every gram of starch is proportionate to roughly 4 calories. Cases of starches are bread, pasta, grain, sugar, potatoes, and rice.

Fats:

The media has totally decimated the notoriety of fats and along these lines when we hear the word we frequently connect it with equivalent words, for example, "terrible". Anyway fats are not all terrible and some fat is important for ideal wellbeing. There are three kinds of fats, soaked, unsaturated and Trans. For the most part trans-fat are terrible and increment your danger of coronary illness. Soaked fats are a bit much awful but rather ought to be restricted to a little percent of your eating regimen. Sustenance's with immersed fats are meat, margarine, grease, cream, and so on. Unsaturated fats have been demonstrated to diminish your danger of creating coronary illness. You can incorporate unsaturated fats into your eating regimen by expending nourishments, for example, avocados, nuts and any sustenance cooked with olive oil.

Caloric Maintenance:

Caloric upkeep is essentially the quantity of calories your body needs in day to look after homeostasis, which is to have no weight put on or weight reduction yet to remain at harmony. Caloric upkeep changes with every person. It might be higher on the off chance that you are more youthful, more dynamic, and have more bulk. Your caloric support will be accomplished through a blend of protein, starches and fats. By and large for new students I suggest a standard 40/40/20 proportion which implies 40% protein, 40% starches and 20% fats. For instance I for the most part eat around

Starvation versus craving

a typical slip-up to make amid an eating regimen is to mistake want starvation. Individuals will regularly feel their stomach snarling and expect that on the off chance that they don't eat soon they will vaporize like a phantom. Well I was joking about the vaporizing, yet individuals will frequently pre-maturely end their quick on the grounds that their stomach was thundering. The commence is that once your body enters starvation mode your digestion rate drops along these lines you will consume less calories and your eating routine will be futile. Anyway that isn't the situation. Concentrates on fasting and digestion has hinted at that the most punctual a lessening in digestion happens following 60 hours and none of the IF projects will make them quick over 24 hours so you won't need to stress over a diminished digestion.

So what do I do about the cravings for food? From individual experience I found that in the event that you simply overlook them and proceed about your day the appetite will leave quickly.

Anyway don't botch hunger with physical agony. In the event that your stomach is in physical agony and really harms then you are accomplishing something incorrectly. If it's not too much trouble counsel a doctor. Fortunately in the event that you take after the IF techniques that I have recorded in part 2 you will never have physical stomach torment.

A fascinating marvel that I find out about yearning is that you can control hunger. Before I began utilizing irregular fasting I use to eat 6 dinners every day. You know the entire "in the event that you eat more you will expand your digestion jabber" which has been demonstrated wrong on the off chance that you were pondering. Amid my six suppers daily eating routine I ordinarily ate at 8:00am. 11:00 are, 2:00pm, 5:00pm, 8:00pm and 11:00pm. So amid the main seven day stretch of discontinuous fasting I would end up hungry around similar circumstances on the grounds that my body was so used to eating at those circumstances. Anyway I disregarded my yearning and by my third seven day stretch of IF my resistance for hunger was gradually dispersing and I could go longer without eating. That as well as I would just feel hungry amid the bolstering window of my discontinuous fasting program. So what's the lesson of the story? You are in the ace of your yearning.

Chapter 2: Intermittent Fasting (IF) Programs

The 24 Hour Fast (24 hour fast once a week)

Advanced by Brad Pillion creator of Eat Stop Eat, the 24 hour quick is a quick that endures a whole day. You will just quick on multi day of the week and on the other

6 days you will eat typically. The 24 hour quick is perspectives fat misfortune in a week by week premise. For instance on the off chance that you regularly eat 2000 calories for every day that is an aggregate of 14,000 calories per week. Presently on the off chance that you subtract multi day then you are down to 12,000 calories. On the off chance that you need to find out about this approach and the science behind it look at Eat Stop Eat.

Who is this approach for?

The 24 hour quick works incredible for apprentices and easygoing calorie counters. It is the most straightforward of the considerable number of projects in light of the fact that there is just a single govern to take after. Individuals who are new to IF should begin with the 24 quick and work their way to the next IF programs if wanted.

Rules

1. Don't eat for 24 hours

Instructions

    1. Pick multi day you might want to quick on

    2. Set the starting time for your quick for instance in the event that you choose that your last dinner ought to be at 8:00pm on Wednesday than you will quick until 8:00pm on Thursday

    3. Be profitable on your quick day and complete your work.

What not to do

• Don't repay by eating more on the other 6 days. On the off chance that you do end up eating more, realize that you have some space for pad. For instance on the off chance that you ate an additional 400 calories on Friday realize that you are still in a shortage of 1600 (2000-400) so don't stress.

• Don't consider nourishment amid your quick. Keep your mind involved.

The Lean gains fast (16/8 hours fast)

This approach was made by fitness coach Mark Berkhan and is prevalent among weight-lifters. The approach incorporates a 16 hour quickly go with an 8 hour ncouraging window. The 8 hour eating window ought to be the same consistently. Dinner recurrence isn't vital as long as you eat amid the 8 hours. The Lean gains quick is done day by day instead of once per week. This approach is exceedingly particular and was outline for measure lifters accordingly it is suggested for ompetitors...

Who is the approach for?

The Lean Gains quick is for competitors and any genuine weight lifter. It isn't suggested for easygoing exercisers or novices because of its intricate arranging.

Rules

. Eating routine ought to be high in protein

. You ought to incorporate fasted (preparing while fasted)

. You should cycle starches (preparing days ought to be high in sugars while off-days are bring down in starches).

. Nourishing windows should be steady.

. On preparing days your post exercise feast ought to be your biggest dinner.

. On non-preparing days your first feast ought to be your biggest dinner.

. Make sure to take some BCAA (branch chain amino acids) previously you repare to guarantee that you don't encounter muscle misfortune amid your fasted reparing.

Instructions

. Decide your 16 hour quick period. In a perfect world you would need the quick to stretch out finished night as you rest. In the event that you put your 16 hour quick amid the time that you are alert then it would imply that your 8 hour encouraging window happens amid the time you rest. For instance if your last supper is at 6:00pm on Tuesday than you would quick until 10:00am on Wednesday. Your encouraging window would be from 10:00am to 6:00pm.

2. When you settled on a fasting period your sustaining window will be the rest of the 8 long stretches of the day

3. Decide a period for preparing. Preferably you would need your preparation period to be simply before you encouraging window with the end goal that you first supper of the day will likewise be your post-preparing feast.

What not to do
• Do not plan your fasting period with the end goal that your encouraging window will be an indistinguishable time from the time you regularly rest.

 Does not neglect to take your BCAAs before you continue with fasted-preparing? Most protein supplements contain BCAAs.

The Warrior Diet (20/4 hour fast)

The warrior eating regimen is a 20 hour quick period took after by a 4 hour nourishing window. Like Lean gains, The Warrior eating regimen is day by day as well. The warrior eating routine was made by Ore Hofmekler and is enlivened by nourishing propensities for Greek warriors and Spartans. With this arrangement you would either quick or eat miniscule measures of sustenance for 18-20 hours. At that point you would devour a lion's share of your every day caloric admission in the rest of the 4-6 hours. In a perfect world you should put your encouraging window close to the finish of the day as it is more helpful for family suppers and after-work instructional courses. The main issue with The Warrior Diet is that attempting to fit your every day caloric admission in one supper can be troublesome. In rundown The Warrior eating routine is essentially a 20 hour quick took after by one huge dinner.

Who is this approach for?

The warrior eating regimen is for individuals who are searching for a passage poin into fasting. This eating routine is extremely adaptable and not as strict as Lean gains. This eating regimen is a most loved for individuals who love to go overboard in calorie thick sustenance (i.e. pizza, burgers, cakes, etc.)The warrior eating routine is an awesome basic eating regimen to fasting. It makes changing to a conventional quick less demanding as it enables you to have little snacks amid the day given that your tidbits need to comprise of products of the soil. In the event that you are hoping to experiment with fasting or get a thought of what fasting is about begin with The Warrior Diet.

Rules

1. Quick for no less than 18-20 hours.

    2. Bites are kept to vegetable and organic products, incidentally a protein shake

    3. Keep your eating regimen high in protein (recollect no less than 1 gram for every pound of bodyweight)

    4. Attempt to meet your every day calorie needs in a single dinner, which means you can enjoy calorie thick nourishment to contact you objective. Well in fact talking it would one say one isn't feast since you have 4 hours to eat what you need to, however let's be realistic what number of individuals is as yet hungry after the primary supper?

Instructions

1. Figure out what supper you need to put you encouraging window around (i.e. breakfast, lunch, supper)

    2. Decide how vast you need you encouraging window to be 4-6 hours is the min and max. Your fasting period will be the rest of the hours in the day.

    3. Choose in the event that you need to eat snacks or complete a total quick amid the day. Keep in mind your tidbits must be either organic products or vegetables and perhaps a protein shake.

What not to do

1. Try not to eat anything calorie thick for snacks, for example, chips, desserts, cakes. Just foods grown from the ground are permitted (infant carrots, spinach

wraps, grapes, apples, and so on).

2. Try not to have any expansive dinners outside of you nourishing window

3. Don't always switch up your one huge feast (i.e. going from supper on multi day to breakfast of the following day) keep it reliable.

Example (warrior diet: dinner)
Mon
7:00am to 5:00pm (assumes 7:00am is   Fasted period
the start of the day)
6:00pm to 10:pm   Feeding Window (mainly Dinner)
11:pm to 6:00   Fasted Period/Sleep

The Alternate Day Fast (36/12 hours fast)

On this program you eat each other day. Essentially you eat in a 12 hour window, say 7:00am to 7:00pm on Monday. At that point you can quick for the rest of Monday and all through Tuesday. On Wednesday you eat again from 7:00am to 7:00pm. Do this process again. Amid your encouraging window you may eat anything you want anyway it is prescribed that you eating regimen predominantly comprise of wholesome nourishment. The other quick eating routine was promoted by Dr. James B. Johnson, if you don't mind bolster him and purchase his book, The Alternate Day Diet, in the event that you wish to know more.

Who is this approach for?

The alternate day diet is suited for the general public i.e. the casual dieter. It is easy to pick up and apply. I would recommend this IF program for beginners as it isn't too strict and it does not have to be used in conjunction with a training program.

Rules

1. Fast for 36 hours.

2. Eat normally during the 12 hour feeding window

3. You may eat anything you like, calorie dense food in moderation of course (unless you are severely behind on your calories and need a boost).

Instructions

1. Determine the time for your 12 hour feeding window. Note most people choose the start time as the time when they first get out of bed.

2. Your fasted period will be the remaining 12 hours of that day plus the next day. You will eat the day after your fasted day.

Chapter 3: Intermittent Fasting (IF) and You

Deciding if Intermittent Fasting (IF) is for you

Irregular fasting isn't for everybody. A few people shed pounds better on a customary eating regimen with general feast recurrence and a few people react better to an IF program. So before you begin any IF program I prescribe you endeavor to quick for one entire day. Correct; simply do whatever it takes not to eat anything for 24 hours. You may discover that you get bothered effortlessly when fasting and choose that fasting isn't for you. You may likewise find that you are additional gainful when you don't need to stress over eating and conclude that you need to experiment with a progress IF program. So to try things out you ought to

1. Quick for one entire day. In the event that your last feast is at 8:00pm on Monday do whatever it takes not to eat until 8.00pm on Tuesday.

Make certain to make a note of how you felt amid the day. Record things like your state of mind, yearning, efficiency and anything you esteem applicable.

I need to attempt Intermittent Fasting (IF)

Okay so you completed a 24 hour quick and conclude that you might want to proceed with discontinuous fasting. So where do you begin? The least demanding path is to choose one of the projects in section 2 and begin from that point.

1. Survey the projects in section 2 and choose which one is most appropriate for your way of life

2. Take after the directions recorded with the program.

3. Keep the quick going until the point that you come to your coveted bodyweight. Note that you can keep the quick going uncertainly or end it at whatever point you need.

4. Make certain to record your advance and alter as needs be.

Outlining your own particular IF program

On the other hand in the event that you don't care for any of the projects in section 2 you can make your own. Anyway I don't prescribe attempting this until the point when you have some involvement with IF. In any case, on the off chance that you do conclude that you need to manufacture your own program here are a few stages to control you.

To start with see that all the IF programs have a couple of things in like manner. Utilize these shared traits as a general rule when planning your own IF program.

• They all contain a fasted period and a bolstering window

• The fasting time frame is for the most part longer than the encouraging window

• Try not to have your fasting period surpass 36 hours in light of the fact that once it does you will begin to lose the advantages of fasting and may encounter really starvation.

So in the event that you needed to plan your own particular IF program.

. In the first place choose how regularly you need to quick (day by day, once per week, each other day).

. At that point choose to what extent you need your quick period to be (36 hours most extreme)

. At that point your encouraging window will naturally be the rest of the hours that you aren't fasting.

. Put your arrangement to activity the following day or the following week.

Tips for Success

Here are a couple of tips to remember while you experiment with IF.

. Begin moderate. Take as much time as is needed and gradually subside into your IF program. Keep in mind you don't need to keep up inflexible adherence. You might need to have a go at fasting once every prior month you have a go at fasting week after week or day by day.

. Trial. Everybody is extraordinary and a cutout program won't work for everybody. Begin with one of the formats and change it to suit you. For instance you may discover that specific sustenance's don't concur with your guts or you may find that you react better to a more drawn out quick. a. Make a speculation

. Test it out

. Report your outcomes

. Modify

. Find. Returning to tip 3 you will find a considerable measure about your body. You will discover things, for example,

The best time for you to eat

The most effortless absorbable nourishment for your body

The best time for you to prepare

• Your caloric upkeep

When you have enough experience you won't ever fear putting on weight again as you'll realize that losing it isn't as hard as everybody made it out to be.

4. Try not to settle what isn't broken. It the eating routine is working and you are getting comes about than allow it to sit unbothered. Notwithstanding if fat misfortune has achieve a level than consider altering. You may need to bring down the calories somewhat more (100 calories less is a decent addition).

5. Expect disappointment. This tip is valid for considerably more than just weight control plans. The fact of the matter is not very many individuals will prevail on their first attempt however what truly matters is your main event a short time later. On the off chance that you attempted IF and didn't make any outcomes than audit what turned out badly and right it. Be that as it may, don't stop following multi week. Give it no less than multi month.

6. Tune in to your body. Our bodies are continually speaking with us. It's simply that a great many people don't know how to decipher the messages. Some normal signals are recorded in the accompanying table.

Positive Cues   Negative Cues

more vitality   Less vitality

Better rest quality   Less rest

Positive state of mind changes (e.g. cheerful, casual, quiet, less dissatisfaction)
Negative state of mind changes (e.g. effectively fractious, baffled, outrage,

Expanded concentration headaches

More beneficial appearance Lack of consideration

7. Sustenance decisions are vital. Keep in mind what I said in part 1 in regards to common sustenance's? If not return and rehash "All are sustenance's square with?

8. The best weight reduction is slowest. Individuals regularly wind up disappointed with eating regimen programs since they aren't seeing quick outcomes. Anyway

abstaining from excessive food intake is a marathon and the best get-healthy plan is the one in which you get more fit in a moderate steady way. Think about the accompanying situations

Situation 1: individual A has been eating less junk food for 2 weeks with an extreme calorie deficiency. Individual A has misfortune 10lbs out of 2 weeks yet now weight reduction has stopped. Affirm, with the goal that individual has figured out how to lose 10lbs yet what amount of that weight was muscle? Furthermore, more imperatively will that individual recover all the weight they lost?

Situation 2: man B has been slimming down for 2 weeks and has figured out how to lose one pound for each week. Anyway the individual proceeds with this pattern for the following year and loses a sum of 52lbs aggregate with negligible muscle misfortune.

To aggregate it up endeavor to be in situation 2. Record your weight week after week and ensure you lose 1 to 2 pounds every week.

9. Be Productive. The quick is the best time to be gainful and complete things. On the off chance that you are always centered on work then the quick would be over before you know it. In any case on the off chance that you lounge around and brood about sustenance, odds are you will break you quick pre-maturely.

10. IF is simply one more part of your life.

This is the most essential tip of every one of them. In the event that like exercise is simply something we consolidate in our life to make life less demanding and more pleasant. On the off chance that makes our life less complex is by expelling our stresses over eating and enables us more opportunity to take a shot at different parts of our life. In the event that irregular fasting causes you worry than quit doing it. In life we as of now have enough wellsprings of stress you needn't bother with another. Keep in mind you don't need to keep up strict adherence to a discontinuous fasting program the center of irregular fasting is, now and then you eat, and in some cases you don't. On the off chance that you can in any event take after that than you will rehearse irregular fasting in its humblest frame.

CHAPTER four: The Health Benefits of Intermittent Fasting (IF)

Another concept for Intermittent Fasting (IF)

Discontinuous fasting is term instituted by the examination world that alludes to deliberately not eating for an expanded timeframe. Trust it or not, people are developmentally adjusted to performing irregular fasts – our predecessors performed broadened fasts at whatever point nourishment was inaccessible, and devoured just when they could get enough sustenance to eat. In any case, in our advanced universe of wealth, purposely fasting for a broadened timeframe is definitely not "typical." Fasting conflicts with each piece of present day life, and is contrary to the abundance-based nourishment culture that we have worked so difficult to make. In our universe of drive-thru food, on-demand nourishment conveyance and 24-hour accommodation stores, picking not to eat sustenance can appear to be odd for sure. I spent my whole graduate profession researching the impacts of irregular fasting in rodents, with a specific end goal to comprehend why fasting is viewed as the best quality level for enhancing one's responsiveness to insulin. Because of this dynamic assemblage of research, countless individuals over the world take part in irregular fasting on a week by week premise, as methods for enhancing their body piece, losing fat mass, shedding pounds or watching a religious occasion. The exploration world has taken an extensive enthusiasm for calorie limitation and irregular fasting, for the express reason for distinguishing cell systems that may impede the maturing procedure. Also, during the time spent concentrate discontinuous fasting, specialists have revealed a clothing rundown of medical advantages that befuddle even the most instructed teachers. In all actuality people have been fasting for a great many years. Present day look into is playing catch-up, keeping in mind the end goal to comprehend why the medical advantages are so noteworthy.

The Health Benefits of Intermittent Fasting (IF)

There is just a single method to build your life expectancy:

decrease your calorie consumption. Confine your calorie allows by 25% and you may add a very long time to your life. Just expressed, there is no pill you can take, no measure of activity you can perform, and no sustenance you can eat that can really make you live more (1– 9). You should simply lessen your sustenance admission, and look as your life span really increments. How does this function? Surprisingly confining your calorie consumption defers the beginning of numerous age-related illnesses, including coronary illness, diabetes, hypertension and growth. More than 75 long stretches of research has revealed some stunning advantages of calorie confinement and irregular fasting, and the outcomes are abridged beneath:

Decreased LDL (the terrible cholesterol) (10,11)

Expanded HDL cholesterol (the great cholesterol)

• Reduced triglycerides

• Reduced pulse

• Reduced aggravation

• Reduced disease chance (tumor development and movement) (12)

• Increased fat consuming and fat misfortune

• Improved body creation

Enhanced Insulin Sensitivity

To the extent glucose digestion is concerned, discontinuous fasting is a flat out goldmine. Irregular fasting is a fantastically ground-breaking instrument for normalizing glucose and enhancing glucose fluctuation.

Aside from work out, discontinuous fasting is the most intense common insulin sensitizer known to man. The particular impacts of irregular fasting on diabetes are recorded here (13– 24):

Lessened fasting blood glucose

• Reduced post-prandial (after feast) blood glucose

• Reduced glucose changeability

• Increased insulin affectability • on a sub-atomic level, for what reason does irregular fasting enhance insulin affectability? Our present understanding channels down to the accompanying fundamentally critical baffle pieces.

Improved Fat Clearance in Muscle and Liver

Insulin obstruction is characterized as the collection in tissues that are not intended to store fat (chiefly the muscle and liver). When you limit admission everything being equal, fat and protein, tissues the whole way across your body must choose the option to consume their put away installed fuel for vitality. When you quick for a broadened timeframe, the fat stores that have aggregated after some time, it turn into the fuel that cells need to work. Subsequently, the extent of the overabundance fat bead gets littler after some time. Strangely, as the measure of the lipid bead in muscle and liver cells diminishes, those cells turn out to be more receptive to insulin. At the end of the day, by diminishing the measure of the fat bead, insulin urns out to be all the more ground-breaking (13– 24).

Leeway of Oxidized Cholesterol Deposits in Blood Vessels

To the extent glucose digestion is concerned, the versatility of your vasculature is as imperative as the soundness of body tissues. Given that glucose and insulin circle in the blood, the less demanding they can cross the dividers of veins the more inconsistent high blood glucose moves toward becoming. Lipid stores collect within mass of veins with age, and after some time these lipid and cholesterol stores end up oxidized. Oxidized stores solidify and frame blood clusters, impeding veins, expanding circulatory strain, solidifying vessel dividers and expanding the hazard for a heart assault.

Studies have demonstrated that calorie confinement and discontinuous fasting are both useful for decreasing these vascular outcomes of maturing, bringing about essened LDL cholesterol, expanded HDL, decreased blood vessel blockage, diminished circulatory strain also, and enhanced transport of glucose and insulin over the vessel dividers.

Consider discontinuous fasting as your one-stop-shop for achieving superb vascular wellbeing, for decreasing cholesterol, diminishing circulatory strain, and verting against vascular entanglements in the long haul. A metabolic triple is whammy without a doubt.

It is safe to say that you are Really Hungry?

Let be honest, we eat when we're feeling forlorn. Also, pitiful

What's more baffled

What's more irate?

Cheerful, confounded, energized. We eat because of our feelings, and this immediate association for the most part brings about… indulging. There are two kinds of craving, what's more, understanding the genuine distinction between them is essential in deciding precisely when to eat nourishment.

Playing out a solitary discontinuous quick is an awesome method to encounter the distinction between our two sorts of yearning: physiological appetite and enthusiastic craving. Physiological craving is the sort of appetite you encounter when your mind, muscles furthermore, inside organs are in a low-energy state. This is the sort of yearning that you

encounter following a requesting exercise. It's the kind of craving you encounter when you have applied noteworthy physical or mental vitality, and need fuel to recharge your vitality needs. Physiological yearning is the flag to consumption sugars, fats, furthermore, protein so as to meet the vitality prerequisites of repairing and developing tissues. Enthusiastic craving is the sort of appetite you encounter when a circumstance or point of view manages your longing to eat. Instead of physiological craving, passionate appetite makes a sentiment of genuine hunger despite the fact that the organic prerequisite for fuel is low or nonexistent.

Understanding the contrast among these sorts of yearning can make a colossal contrast to your general wellbeing. Do you eat when you're just physiologically hungry? Do you eat when you're candidly ravenous? Do you eat in the two circumstances? Playing out a solitary irregular quick can enable you to decide the contrast between the two quickly.

Test Intermittent Fasting (IF) Regimens

Regardless of how you cut it, irregular fasting isn't only bravo, it's GREAT for you. Notwithstanding the physical advantages depicted above, deliberately confining sustenance allow notwithstanding for a solitary 24-hour period can be very testing, and encourages you build up a genuine autonomy from nourishment.

There are unlimited stages of discontinuous fasting regimens, so I'll exhibit as it were the ones that are achievable and gloat noteworthy here and now benefits. There is no sense in doing irregular fasting if the immediate advantage takes months or years to accomplish. Fortunate for you, playing out a solitary discontinuous quick is a fun ordeal that can have a discernible and quantifiable effect in your wellbeing.

The most achievable discontinuous fasting regimen is the once-per-week 24-hour discontinuous quick, as portrayed beneath:

The Weekly 24-Hour Intermittent fast
similarly as the name suggests, pick multi day of the week and don't eat.

Sunday .Monday ,Tuesday ----→Eat Normally-

Wednesday------============- → 24-Hour Fast
Thursday Friday Saturday ------- .>Eat Normally

The Twice Per Week 24-Hour Intermittent Fast

Like the week by week 24-hour discontinuous quick, this one includes a second 24-hour time of fasting for special reward.

Sunday Tuesday Wednesday Friday Saturday--→ Eat Normally

Monday Thursday -→ 24-Hour Fast

The Magic of Negative Energy Balance

Every one of the above discontinuous fasting regimens point by point above, amid the period of fasting you enter negative vitality adjust in which your rate of vitality consumption surpasses your rate of vitality admission. As it were, you are losing vitality all through the fasting time frame. You may believe that it's conceivable to eat twice much nourishment. Instantly thereafter, so as to make up for the measure of nourishment that you didn't eat amid your quick.
In actuality be that as it may, it is exceptionally hard to eat enough to make up for your fasting period, which brings about a continuation of negative vitality adjust

even after the fasting period is finished.

Negative vitality adjust is precisely the shrouded "enchantment" of the discontinuous quick.

Rather than calorie limitation in which you are ravenous each day, performing irregular fasts on a predefined day of the week permits you a psychological and physical break from fasting, which is fundamental for long haul achievement.

The 24-Hour Intermittent Fast
Let's assume that you do a Thursday fast. Here is an example 24-hour protocol:
7pm Wednesday:
Eat your last meal of the day
Drink 500 mills (2 cups) of water
Go to sleep
8pm Wednesday:
START FAST
8am Thursday:
Drink 1 L (4 cups) of water, or…
Drink 250 mills (1 cup) of green tea
12pm Thursday:
Drink 1 L (4 cups) of water, or…
Drink 250 mills (1 cup) of green tea
3pm Thursday:
Drink 1 L (4 cups) of water, or…
Drink 250 mills, (1 cup) green tea.
7pm Thursday:
UNOFFICIALLY END FAST
Eat a *small* dinner before bed, complete with plenty of real carbohydrates
Drink 500 mills (2 cups) of water
7am Friday:
OFFICIALLY END FAST
Return to your normal eating schedule

Meal Time Liquid Options

2-3 Cups of Water
Drink 2-3 cups of water at meal time to help distend
Your stomach and "fake" the feeling of being full.
When your stomach distends, it sends a signal to your Brain, it which can curb
your feelings of hunger.

1-2 Cups of Green Tea
Drink 1-2 cups of green tea at meal time, to help curb, your feelings of hunger.
Green tea can often act as an
Appetite suppressant to curb your feelings of hunger,
And it does it remarkably well.

Tips and Strategies for Easing Through the Intermittent Fast

-The green tea is not essential to fasting, but it can make the experience
Easy, Green tea can act as an appetite suppressant and curb, your feelings of
Hunger
- Drinking water in particular helps to mitigate feelings of hunger by filling your
Stomach. This sends a signal to your brain and often results in you feeling less
Hungry .
- Be aware of your body cues. Feeling stressed out or "upset" during your fast?
Relax.
- Take a few deep breaths, and pay close attention — this is what true hunger
Can feel like
- Have healthy food (lean protein, veggies, etc.) in the house and ready to go
During you "break" the fast on Sunday night with a small meal.

-Also, having healthy food in the house is good insurance that you won't binge
The following day when you return to normal eating

The Modified 24-Hour Intermittent Fast
Why do a Modified Intermittent Fast?

For some people, performing a full 24-hour fast is very difficult. Especially for people with diabetes, fasting for extended periods of time can increase the risk for Hypoglycemia (low blood glucose), so it is very important to counteract this risk by having food on hand. If you fall into one of these categories, consider performing a modified 24-hour fast:

-You have type 1 diabetes
-You have type 2 diabetes
-You are prone to hypoglycemia (low blood glucose)
-You have a very difficult time concentrating when hungry
-You experience violent mood swings when fasting

What is Hypoglycemia (Low Blood Glucose)?

The main reason why it is difficult to perform a true 24-hour intermittent fast for Some people is because when you consume no calories for an extended period of Time, your brain can often becomes starved for fuel, resulting in any of the following feelings:

☐ Mood swings
☐ Frustration
☐ Anger
☐ Inability to concentrate
☐ Shaky hands
☐ Slurred speech

How is a Modified Intermittent Fast Different than a True?

Intermittent Fast

The major difference between a true and modified intermittent fast is the amount
Of Calories that you take in at meal time. In a true intermittent fast, you consume
Calories at meal times, whereas in a modified intermittent fast, you consume a
small
Number of calories (about 100-200 calories) at meal time. Even with a small intake
Of calories, you still get some exceptional health benefits!

Example Protocol
Let's assume that you do a Thursday fast. Here is an example 24-hour modified
Protocol:
7pm Wednesday:
Eat your last meal of the day
Drink 500 mills (2 cups) of water
Go to sleep
4pm Wednesday:
START FAST
8am Thursday:
Drink 1 L (4 cups) of water, or…
Drink 250 mills (1 cup) of vegetable juice
12pm Thursday:
Drink 1 L (4 cups) of water, or…
Drink 250 mills (1 cup) of green tea
4pm Thursday:
Drink 1 L (4 cups) of water, or…
Eat a vegetable snack or 1-2 pieces of fruit
7pm Thursday:
UNOFFICIALLY END FAST
Eat a *small* dinner before bed, complete with plenty of real carbohydrates
Drink 500 mills (2 cups) of water
7am Friday:
OFFICIALLY END FAST
Return to your normal eating schedule
100-200 Calorie Meal Options

1 Cup of Vegetable Juice
Drink 1 8 oz. cup of vegetable juice, made from any
Combination of tomatoes, beets, celery, carrots,
Cucumbers, mint, parsley, arugula, kale
1-2 Pieces of Your Favorite Fruit
Eat 1-2 piece of your favorite fruit (banana, apple,
Pear, persimmon, orange, a handful of berries etc.)
1-2 Servings of Vegetables
Eat 1-2 servings of vegetables (cauliflower, tomatoes,
Carrots, broccoli, Brussels sprouts, okra etc.)
8-10 of Your Favorite Nuts
Eat 8-10 nuts (cashews, walnuts, almonds, Brazil nuts
Etc.)
A Small Bowl of Salad
Eat a small salad containing 1 serving of vegetables
(Salad base is made from any combination of cabbage,
Spinach, lettuce, arugula, kale)

Conclusion:

 Intermittent fasting benefits are robust and easy to experience. All it takes is a
willingness to skip a few meals. Intermittent fasting is an easy way to burn excess
fat and is believed to be an incredible tool for preventing chronic disease and
improving longevity, strength and overall health. On the off chance that I needed t
entirety up irregular fasting in a couple of principles I would state this

1. Eat in some cases yet not constantly

2. When you do eat, pick the most nutritious nourishments

3. Enjoy your most loved nourishments once in a while

4. Make sure to work out.

5. "Grin, inhale, and go gradually." – Thick Nhat HanH

References

1. Berardi, J. M., Scott-Dixon, K., & Green, N. (2012).*Experiments with intermittent fasting*. Precision Nutrition. Retrieved from http://www.precisionnutrition.com/intermittent-fasting

2. Romaniello, J. (2010). http://www.romanfitnesssystems.com/blog/intermittent-fasting-101/ *Intermittent Fasting (IF) 101*. Retrieved from

3. Romaniello, J. (2012). http://www.romanfitnesssystems.com/blog/intermittent-fasting-201/ *Intermittent Fasting (IF) 201*. Retrieved from

4. Berkhan, M. (2010, April 14). *The leangains guide*. Retrieved from http://www.leangains.com/2010/04/leangains-guide.html

5. Park, M. (2010, Nov 08). Twinkie diet helps nutrition professor lose 27 pounds. Retrieved from http://www.cnn.com/2010/HEALTH/11/08/twinkie.diet.professor/index.html

6. Freediet.com daily caloric calculator. (n.d.). Retrieved from http://www.freedieting.com/tools/calorie_calculator.htm

References

1. Guarente L. Calorie restriction and SIR2 genes--towards a mechanism. Mech Ageing Dev. 2005 Sep;126(9):923–8.
2. Houthoofd K, Vanfleteren JR. The longevity effect of dietary restriction in Caenorhabditis elegans. Exp Gerontol. 2006 Oct;41(10):1026–31.
3. Partridge L, Piper MDW, Mair W. Dietary restriction in Drosophila. Mech Ageing Dev. 2005 Sep;126(9):938–50.
4. Ramsey JJ, Harper ME, Weindruch R. Restriction of energy intake, energy expenditure, and aging. Free Radic Biol Med. 2000 Nov 15;29(10):946–68.
5. Colman RJ, Anderson RM, Johnson SC, Kastman EK, Kosmatka KJ, Beasley TM,
et al. Caloric Restriction Delays Disease Onset and Mortality in Rhesus Monkeys. Science. 2009 Jul 10;325(5937):201–4.
6. Das SK, Gilhooly CH, Golden JK, Pittas AG, Fuss PJ, Cheatham RA, et al. Longterm
effects of 2 energy-restricted diets differing in glycemic load on dietary adherence, body composition, and metabolism in CALERIE: a 1-y randomized controlled trial. Am J Clin Nutr. 2007 Apr 1;85(4):1023–30.
7. Mattison JA, Roth GS, Lane MA, Ingram DK. Dietary restriction in aging nonhuman primates. Interdiscip Top Gerontol. 2007;35:137–58.
8. Anderson RM, Shanmuganayagam D, Weindruch R. Caloric restriction and aging: studies in mice and monkeys. Toxicol Pathol. 2009 Jan;37(1):47–51.
9. Masoro EJ. Caloric restriction and aging: an update. Exp Gerontol. 2000

May;35(3):299–305.

10. Fontana L, Meyer TE, Klein S, Holloszy JO. Long-term calorie restriction is highly effective in reducing the risk for atherosclerosis in humans. Proc Natl Acad Sci U S A. 2004 Apr 27;101(17):6659–63.

11. Roth GS, Ingram DK, Lane MA. Caloric Restriction in Primates and Relevance to Humans. Ann N Y Acad Sci. 2001;928(1):305–315.

12. Pallavi R, Giorgio M, Pelicci PG. Insights into the beneficial effect of caloric/ dietary restriction for a healthy and prolonged life. Front Physiol [Internet]. 2012 Aug 9 [cited 2014 Apr 14];3. Available from: http://www.ncbi.nlm.nih.gov/pmc/articles/PMC3429088/

13. Larson-Meyer DE, Heilbronn LK, Redman LM, Newcomer BR, Frisard MI, Anton S, et al. Effect of Calorie Restriction With or Without Exercise on Insulin Sensitivity, β-Cell Function, Fat Cell Size, and Ectopic Lipid in Overweight Subjects. Diabetes Care. 2006 Jun 1;29(6):1337–44.

14. Heilbronn LK, de Jonge L, Frisard MI, DeLany JP, Larson-Meyer DE, Rood J, et al. Effect of 6-month calorie restriction on biomarkers of longevity, metabolic adaptation, and oxidative stress in overweight individuals: a randomized controlled trial. JAMA J Am Med Assoc. 2006 Apr 5;295(13):1539–48.

15. Weiss EP, Holloszy JO. Improvements in body composition, glucose tolerance, and insulin action induced by increasing energy expenditure or decreasing energy intake. J Nutr. 2007 Apr;137(4):1087–90.

16. Dean DJ, Cartee GD. Brief dietary restriction increases skeletal muscle glucose transport in old Fischer 344 rats. J Gerontol A Biol Sci Med Sci. 1996 May;51(3):B208-213.

17. Anson RM, Guo Z, Cabo R de, Iyun T, Rios M, Hagepanos A, et al. Intermittent fasting dissociates beneficial effects of dietary restriction on glucose metabolism and neuronal resistance to injury from calorie intake. Proc Natl Acad Sci. 2003 May 13;100(10):6216–20.

18. McCurdy CE, Cartee GD. Akt2 Is Essential for the Full Effect of Calorie Restriction on Insulin-Stimulated Glucose Uptake in Skeletal Muscle. Diabetes. 2005 May 1;54(5):1349–56.

19. Cartee GD, Dean DJ. Glucose transport with brief dietary restriction: heterogenous responses in muscles. Am J Physiol - Endocrinol Metab. 1994 Jun 1;266(6):E946–52.

20. Cartee GD, Kietzke EW, Briggs-Tung C. Adaptation of muscle glucose transport

with caloric restriction in adult, middle-aged, and old rats. Am J Physiol - Regul Integr Comp Physiol. 1994 May 1;266(5):R1443–7.
21. Davidson RT, Arias EB, Cartee GD. Calorie restriction increases muscle insulin
action but not IRS-1-, IRS-2-, or phosphotyrosine-PI 3-kinase. Am J Physiol - Endocrinol Metab. 2002 Feb 1;282(2):E270–6.
22. Dean DJ, Brozinick JT, Cushman SW, Cartee GD. Calorie restriction increases cell surface GLUT-4 in insulin-stimulated skeletal muscle. Am J Physiol - Endocrinol Metab. 1998 Dec 1;275(6):E957–64.
23. McCurdy CE, Davidson RT, Cartee GD. Brief calorie restriction increases Akt2
phosphorylation in insulin-stimulated rat skeletal muscle. Am J Physiol - Endocrinol Metab. 2003 Oct 1;285(4):E693–700.
24. Wing RR, Blair EH, Bononi P, Marcus MD, Watanabe R, Bergman RN. Caloric
Restriction Per Se Is a Significant Factor in Improvements in Glycemic Control and Insulin Sensitivity During Weight Loss in Obese NIDDM Patients. Diabetes Care. 1994 Jan 1;17(1):30–6.

www.ingramcontent.com/pod-product-compliance
Lightning Source LLC
Chambersburg PA
CBHW051404250726
48656CB00006B/2265